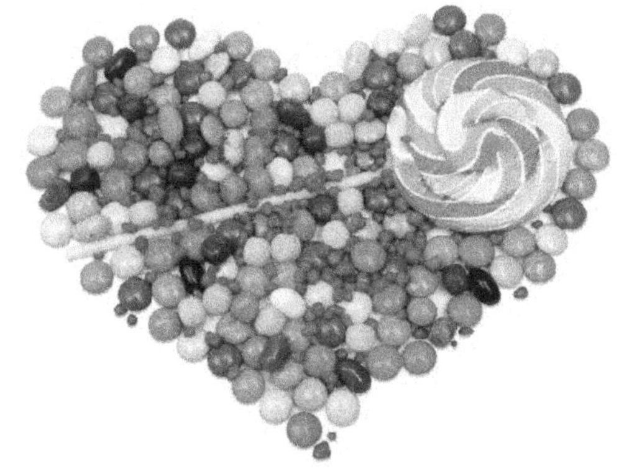

Don's Heart

Medical Marvels Happen at All Ages

By Don Sivertsen

Dear Reader:
This book is about my heart and from my heart to you.
Although I know nothing about medicine and have no
intention of influencing anyone to do as I did in any way, I do
hope my story encourages those who are discouraged about
health issues in their later years. I'm 90 now (2017) and had
these wonderful experiences this year! Again, I know
everyone and every situation is different. I hope for all of you
that you have as good a doctor as I do and that you will see
and listen to that doctor.
With a full and grateful heart,
Don Sivertsen

AWARENESS

One day, I went to the library and saw three people sitting at a table in the lobby. I asked if they were giving health tests, and they said, "Yes. Would you like us to check your blood pressure?" Why not? I thought.

A woman put the cuff on my arm and I felt the pressure as it tightened. My blood pressure was ok, she assured me, but I had an irregular heartbeat. She wrote on my test that I should see my doctor immediately.

I shrugged it off, told her it didn't surprise me as I'm ninety years old. People don't live forever. I was worried, though and didn't tell my family doctor about it for two months. Then he gave me an electro cardiogram test.

"Don! I'm referring you to a cardiologist."

Now, I really was worried and made an appointment immediately, and, as you'll see, this was the right thing to do.

These health stations with their volunteers are all around us, even at the summer street fairs, available to all. The free basic tests can make us aware of health conditions and warn of problems. I'm certainly glad I stopped that day and had my pulse and blood pressure checked.

I SHOULD HAVE HEART PROCEDURES MORE OFTEN

The idea that I will not be able to do very much after my heart procedure has given me impetus to get busy painting a panel on my house, hiring a carpenter to do some work for me. Wash all my clothes so I will have clean sheets. Stock up on bread and TV chicken pies—enough for at least a week. I plan maybe to sort and organize my papers. Clean off my tables. I do want to go to the Fisherman's Festival on the twenty-third, only three days after my trip to the hospital. I may have to have someone take me there.

This is Sunday, and I have to work on filling my yard waste container for Tuesday. I'll be fasting for Wednesday when my niece will take me to the hospital. I may have to stay overnight. I'll bring a change of underwear, my toothbrush, my radio, a tablet, a pen, and my cell phone so I can call my friends to let them know I'm still among the living. Hospitals worry me, make me more active to get everything done. Let's do it more often, Hospital.

ONLY THREE DAYS LEFT

On Wednesday, I go in to the Virginia Mason Medical Center for a heart procedure. I will go in at 10 am and out at 6 pm, then back home. Will I be ok? I think so. I think the real danger is possibly bleeding afterward. The irregular heartbeat may be corrected. I could live years longer in good health.

This is what the reason is for this heart procedure. It may reduce the possibility of having a stroke. I made my decision. I would like to keep active, live in my old house, drive, and continue to write. I would like to publish another book, sort out all my papers, organize them and then finish my book, publish it…then retire in luxury on the proceeds. Maybe I better take all my friends on a goodbye cruise to Alaska or the Caribbean. Maybe six people in all. Wouldn't that be fun. A one-week trip on a cruise with some of my good friends.

A DAY TO REMEMBER

September 20, 2017 — this was a big day for me. I had been planning and anticipating it for several weeks. I was going to the hospital for a heart procedure that would help my heart. This procedure is called Catheter Ablation. I was able to go home the same day. All went well. We called my sister Carol (sixteen years younger than I), in Albuquerque New Mexico to let her know I was all right. We asked her husband where Carol was, so I could give her my good news. "She is in the hospital," he said. Carol had fallen and hit her head on the shower glass. "She is all right now and will be going home soon." I found out later she had been under observation for three days and had been tested for a possible heart problem. The words I heard from my sister were very familiar to me. She had been tested and told of a possible procedure that sounded like the same as what I had on the same day. Now isn't that a coincidence…or maybe it was just having similar genes?

That same day I heard my first wife (the mother of my only son) died and a good friend's father also died. September 20, 2017 is a day I'll never forget.

MY HEART PROCEDURE IS OVER

I think I am better. I can tie my shoes now without losing my breath. Take it easy, Don, for the next few days, I tell myself. I am driving again and spent the whole day with friends at the Annual Fisherman's Festival, something I didn't want to miss. I'm back on schedule again on my Sunday morning round trip to Bremerton. This is one of my favorite places to write. The surroundings are tranquilizing: birds, water, a friendly Washington ferry boat crew making it a wonderful experience. I get to sit and contemplate what is going on in my little world. I ride on one of the new ferry boats with very little vibration. We just glide along so effortlessly. I have a full week ahead.

This is the way I like it: keeping busy.

CARDIAC ABLATION

This is what I had, a heart procedure to stop an unwanted electrical circuit. I was in at ten am and out at ten pm, all in one day. Everything went well. I finally was allowed to eat at four pm. Oh, it tasted so good—codfish with a side of green peas and a slice of butter on top. For some unknown reason, every time the doctor zapped my heart with energy, I felt it in my sore right shoulder…but not in my heart. My shoulder ached, a normal reaction I was told. I feel better already, I could tie my shoes today without losing my breath.

Patti took my picture in the hospital, surrounded by hospital gear. I thought it was hilarious. We were told not to laugh—it might cause my puncture to bleed. When we were ready to leave, the nurse called for a wheelchair and my friends took me home.

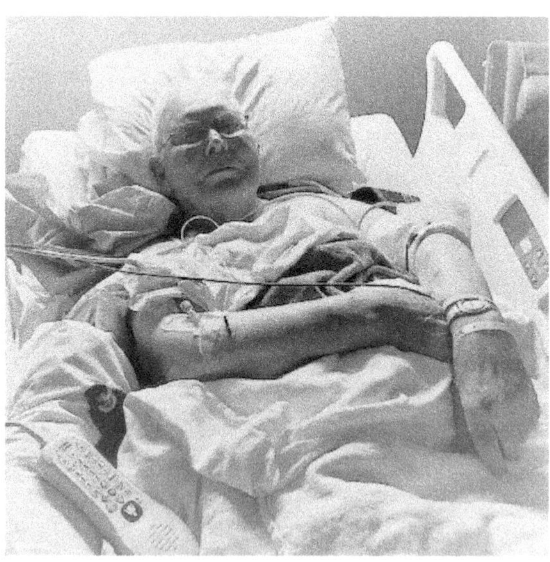

ABLATION

This procedure took care of a problem in my heart — an electrical circuit in my heart that didn't belong there. I had no idea how long I had it. The procedure took two and a half hours. I had to lie still on my back for another six or seven hours before I was released to go home. I call it just a ninety-year tune up for an old man. These doctors today can do almost anything.

When I talk to people about the heart procedure, I just had, others come up with similar stories, but the stories are all somewhat different. These people survived heart surgery and procedures. I would not even know unless I was told. One person has a pig valve, another had a leaking heart that was sewed up. It's remarkable what the medical profession can do today. I had a problem I wasn't even aware I had. Now, I have a normal heart, I am told. Medicine can heal.

LIFE

Maybe my life has been extended with the improvement in my heart. I better appreciate this, to do more with my writing and my lifestyle. I think three or four years more could be possible. Will I be able to drive, maybe? I know many people who had heart procedures, all were different, and they are still living. It might be the attitude. I did it to see if I could improve my health. I already feel better. I'm having a slight improvement in mobility. Doing yard work. I'll know more on Thursday after I see my doctor about my 90-year-old tune up.

MY FAVORITE BUFFET

Today I ate at my favorite buffet. I eat here all the time. Each person takes the ladle or tongs, picking out the food to put on their plate. There was a pretty lady with long flowing black hair in front of me. She was taking her time, so much time I could contemplate…will she pick out the shrimp, the cauliflower, or the Brussel sprouts? She was so slow; maybe she was doing it to annoy me or to get my attention. I didn't mind too much because I was secretly admiring her from behind, while I waited. When she was ready to move on…suddenly, she turned to look me in the eye and said, "Here is the spoon." A thought came to me as I took the spoon from her hand, *I think I'm in love*, but just for a moment…I felt a spark from my heart that made me feel so good. Maybe that heart procedure did some good after all!

Speedy recovery!!
Like Show more reactions
· Reply · September 20 at 7:39pm

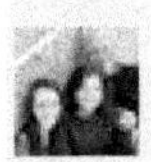

Marlene Koltin Thank you for posting this, Patti. How long will he be there? Up for visitors?
Like Show more reactions
· Reply · September 20 at 8:13pm

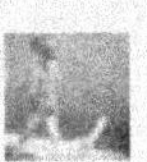

Tanja Jinx Pineda Hugs!!!!!!!
Like Show more reactions
· Reply · September 20 at 8:20pm

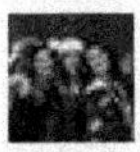

Patti Lozano Hopes to be home late tonight.
Like Show more reactions
· Reply ·
22
· September 20 at 8:27pm

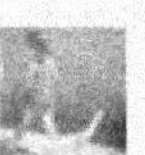

Tanja Jinx Pineda Please give him a hug from me. He was a sweetie when I once lived in Seattle.
Like Show more reactions
· Reply · September 20 at 8:31pm

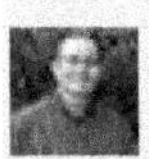

John Roberts He told me he was having a procedure on his heart. He didn't give the impression it was a big deal. Good to know.
Like Show more reactions
· Reply ·
11
· September 20 at 9:48pm

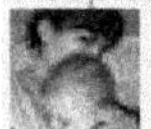

Beth Seren Get well soon 🤍🤍🤍
Like Show more reactions

· Reply · September 20 at 10:36pm

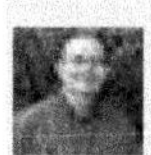

John Roberts Look at those cheekbones. I wish I will look so good if I am in a hospital bed! And no wrinkles, too.
Like Show more reactions
· Reply ·
22
· September 21 at 7:28am

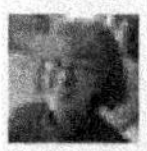

Maryallene Arsanto Feel better, Don! Hope you're home soon.
Like Show more reactions
· Reply ·
22
· September 21 at 7:44am

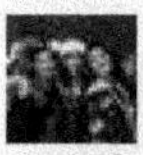

Patti Lozano Don is home and doing well!
Like Show more reactions
· Reply ·
325
· September 21 at 9:29am

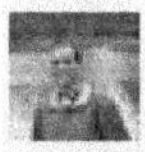

Omar Al Obiedy Wish you a fast recovery, Don.
Like Show more reactions
· Reply ·
22
· September 21 at 6:42pm · Edited

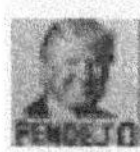

Rick Pannemann Just bumped into Don at the Fisherman's Festival. Looking good!
Like Show more reactions
· Reply ·
44
· September 23 at 3:41pm

WHEN DID I START WRITING?

I attended Bellevue Junior College while I was working night shift when I was 56 years old. I took a karate class. Oh, I might as well take a bonehead English class while I'm there. We had a great teacher and less than ten students in the class. We wrote stories and read them out loud in the class. The stories were very interesting, and I learned a lot in this class. When the term was over, our teacher announced we had done so well and he was so proud of us that he'd given all of us an A in English 101, which did give us a credit for the class.

Since I had passed English, I continued for two years and received a two-year Associate of Arts degree.

Our instructor had told us how important it was to continue writing, do some writing every day. When you write to solve a problem, the letter gets attention, much more than a telephone call. I never forgot this — it brings results. So, this is how and when I took up writing and still continue to do so, thanks to the English teacher I once had.

I WENT TO A WEDDING

It was yesterday. A hundred people attended. Location: north of Everett where the ground had once been a strawberry field. The place had a lot of parking space. Today, this is a where you can have a large wedding or plan a huge one for someone else.

My niece's daughter has two girls, eight and ten years old, the groom has two boys about the same ages. This is to be a big family affair that had been planned for about a year. Everyone was dressed up. I wore what I felt comfortable in, my khaki Docker pants and a clean shirt. I didn't feel out of place even though many wore suits.

I enjoyed the day. After the wedding, we had food buffet style. I'm familiar with this. Your eyes can be bigger than your stomach, so I ate conservatively and celebrated with two glasses of water and the diabetic pill I'd brought with me. I went home early before the party was over without having a taste of the wedding cake, as it was already past my eight o'clock bedtime. This was a day to remember. I could see the joy my sister was having. The women became very emotional at the wedding. Yes, weddings are all right: an opinion I overheard shared by some of the other men, when they were asked.

MY MANY HATS

I always wear a hat when I go out. I don't feel fully dressed without one. I try to protect my eyes from the sun when I am driving and the glare from the oncoming lights at night. I do have my favorite hat but I can't always find it. I grab any hat I can find. Each one of my hats carry a symbol or a message. When I go out in public I'm asked were you in the army WW2 or Vietnam? I thought he was a panhandler, so I looked straight ahead making no eye contact. Later, I found I was wearing the disabled veterans hat—the one I received on my birthday. Another hat the Missouri hat brings the question, "Were you in the navy?" No, I bought it when the ship was in Bremerton. When I wear this one people want to know if I worked for the Washington ferry system. No, a deckhand gave it to me—the workers consider me an honorary passenger because I take a round trip every Sunday without fail. Yes, there is my retired United Airlines hat that is true, and I even met a man who worked with me at the same time. My favorite hat is the one I wear at night. My red stocking that I can't sleep without. It is the hat I wear most often though, of course, no one ever sees me in that because it's the one I wear at night! A hat retains my body heat at night.

Wearing my many hats, protects my eyes and above all they all act as security blankets.

JUST LAST YEAR

I went to get a fishing license. The clerk at the sporting goods store asked me for my name and social security number. "No way," I answered. We have been warned never to give out your SS number to a stranger."
"No fishing license then," he replied.
So at 89, I can't even go fishing or get a fishing license, just watch others. Maybe this is meant to be: My fishing days are over. The state knows what is the best for me.

SHORT PANTS

I really noticed this last week at my 9:30 am meeting on Saturday. I counted about five men who were wearing shorts. This isn't very attractive to look at when you are watching a speaker — old men with hairy legs. I have suggested this before to one whose appearance I was trying to improve. "Wear long pants anytime you get up in front of an audience to speak."

Apparently, my advice just went in one ear and out the other. When you are an evaluator at a Toastmaster contest, a checklist gives about 10 percent for appearance to the person you evaluate. We should practice making a good appearance whenever getting in front of an audience.

I'M 89 TODAY

Sometimes I didn't think I would make it this far. I think I'll set a new goal now. I'll try to reverse those numbers and change them to 98. That is only ten years away. I always set my goals high. If I reach it, fine. With the recent progress made in medicine and with all the pills I take to keep my blood tests near normal, who knows? The odds might be with me. I'm retired living alone. I don't have any stress except what I do to myself like insisting on climbing ladders and then falling occasionally. I have always been able to get up again.

I think that taking several prescribed pills and vitamins has helped me. I go to see my doctor once every three months. He has watched me recover from many illnesses. I even had whooping cough after I retired.

I break all the rules on my diet at least one time every day. I like to have a simple dessert vanilla ice cream with some chocolate syrup and crushed nuts on top.

My only exercise is mowing the lawn and walking around in the store while shopping for groceries. Sometimes, I go to the hot tub, but that isn't really exercise.

I do have a social life. I belong to two toastmaster clubs and two writing classes. I have good neighbors that stop and talk to me once in a while. One is a captain for an airline and tells me about his latest trip. Another friend is a builder who constructs houses. I like to follow the progress he makes while he builds a house. He always has time to talk to me. It's amazing the talents that people have, the diversification of how each person I know makes a living. I always wanted to be independent. Now, at 89 and after 23 years of retirement, all I can say is, it has been a good life.

HOME ALONE

I love to poke around in old torn clothes. I find them comfortable. I can do a project around the house, maybe like painting. It won't worry me if I splash a little paint around and get some on my clothes. That goes also for working on a lawn mower or a bicycle, or just poking around out in the garage. Every once in a while, I don't want to change my clothes. I go just as I am.... I'm only going to the hardware store. It doesn't matter if I'm watching the news on TV or washing the dishes or cooking. The phone rings occasionally. It might be somebody wanting to clean my rugs or to buy my house. It isn't for sale. Oh, it's that Internet computer again, kicking out my age. We'll just keep calling him and sending him letters.

It won't do them any good. He just pokes around the house in his old clothes.

If someone tries to buy my property, I tell him, you'll have to talk to my sister in New Mexico. She has my power of attorney. I can't sign anything. I'm 88 Years old, you know.

RENTERS

I once had a sideline. I owned two other houses and rented
them out. I planned on doing this until the houses were
paid for, then retire when I got old. It didn't work out like I
planned. I would get calls from the renters all the time: The
toilet doesn't flush; there is an odor under the house; the
furnace doesn't work, or the house is cold. Then when it
was time to pay the rent, it was never on time. When the
renters were getting ready to move, I would be on the alert.
Renters have a habit of grabbing anything they can, even
the light bulbs from the sockets. It was partly my fault for
not screening them and not asking for a damage deposit. It
didn't work out at all. I had to work all the time on my
projects and try to hang on to what I owned in the house,
then clean, paint, and look for new renters. I wasn't meant
to be a landlord.
Now I know it.

SUNBURN IN SEATTLE

I parked my car in front of a doughnut shop. The window was open, the sun was out. This was a hot summer day. I fell asleep. I don't know for how long…maybe two and a half hours. I was aware that my hand and my arm were warm. In the past week, my hand had swollen, my skin was red and hot. I was going to go blame it on my new medication. Should I tell my doctor? Then it dawned on me. I had received a severe maybe a third-degree sunburn. I tried to cook my arm under the hot sun in Seattle. The solution is to wear long sleeve shirts and button them up before I go to sleep.

MY TEACHER WILL BE MOVING

I must get busy on my books. Ariele is the key to me
publishing my books. I could not have done it without her
help, without her skill and knowledge of publishing,
editing, and her follow through determination. This means
get on with it, Don. I don't mind typing. My health has
stabilized. I feel good. My heart treatment is over. Now I can
concentrate on what is in my heart: writing stories, self-
publishing. Share some of my thoughts so I can share some
of my life experiences, successes and failures.

With a positive attitude, failure can be turned around. I
really believe this. Don Sivertsen's stories attest to that.
When you are down, get up and try again. Failure can lead
to great success. Just believe in yourself.

I WENT THROUGH A RED LIGHT

It was one of those turning lights, with four cars in front of me. They turned on the green, then on amber. I thought I could make it, then it turned red, and I went through.

This was a big mistake. The big police car behind me was flashing its lights. I pulled over. I had been caught.

I learned when I was younger and getting a ticket (now and then), just comply, show them your credentials. Do whatever, the officer wants.

I showed him my driver's license, registration, and an insurance card, showing I was paid up for this year. I was a little nervous. I showed him my papers, but could not find my PEMCO insurance card, just an old receipt with PEMCO on it.

He talked on his radio, my driver's license in his hand. I had a perfect driving record. "This is not a ticket to go on your record."

I'll get an insurance card and keep it with me at all times…just for insurance…in case I'm stopped again.

FISHERMAN'S FESTIVAL

I try to go every year. It lasts only one day in September, always on a Saturday. The weather has always been good. This festival has something for everybody. Art projects for the children, a stage for all to watch. I always enjoy the reptile man sharing the stories about reptiles. He showed us an alligator, a turtle, and a lot of snakes.

My friend and my niece took a boat trip down the canal to the Fremont Bridge, then it turned around and took us to the Government Locks and back to the festival. We topped that off with a generous portion of alder cooked salmon and corn on the cob.

COFFEE SHOP

Sitting in a new coffee shop for me. I can sit and sip my coffee, look across the street and see the place where I lived when I was a little boy. It brings back memories of my mother, father, and little sister, Lorraine. We lived in one of the two upper apartments that was above the then Petersons grocery store. To the south is a barber shop. I remember when my father took me in for my first haircut. The barber had a board that he placed on top of the barber chair armrests. Then he put me on top of the board, so I could see around as he cut my hair. That was about eighty-five years ago, when I was around five years old.

I thought, *my birthday is coming up. I need a haircut. Why not get my next haircut here*? It will be maybe my first haircut and maybe my last. I will look good for my birthday party.

When I told the lady barber what I could remember, she went over to the wall and pulled out the board they use today when cutting a child's hair. I was a little disappointed. It wasn't the same board I sat on when I was a child. Nevertheless, I had my first haircut and maybe my last there—when I was ninety.

CARING PEOPLE

A good meal, a good night's sleep, can make you feel great. The next morning, everything looks better and can get me off to a good start. A call from a friend and invitation to come over for crackers and cheese — these hit the spot.

Then, I went home to work on my yard waste bin for tomorrow. I felt hot, working with the sun on my back.

My neighbor came by on her bicycle. She helped me do my yard work. It is always easier when two people are working at it. In no time, we had filled the yard waste container. I appreciate my good friends. I seem to be surrounded by people like these two — always willing to go out of their way to make a task easier for me and to let me know they care.

I really appreciate all who make an old man feel important. All that have done so much for me. I give my gratitude to my friends.

About the Author:

Don Sivertsen's first book, *Laughs, Luck & Life* is about an earlier Medical Marvel he experienced. Regaining his ability to speak, think, and write after a stroke, the author presents a uniquely life-affirming series of funny and/or poignant anecdotes characterized by their humble yet self-confident messages. His words—gained by accessing the "spare, unused brain cells" that weren't damaged—are a bright ray of hope served up as warmhearted humor and sprinkled with some modestly offered advice.
Link to *Laughs, Luck & Life*
https://www.amazon.com/dp/B01IFN4DD8.

About the Editor:

Ariele Huff has 20 books of her own on Amazon and specializes in helping others create eBooks and publish-on-demand paperbacks. Her publishing brands are Candy Bar Books and Band-Aid Books. Editor of a dozen magazines and periodicals and hundreds of books, Huff leads ongoing writing groups, teaches at Washington State colleges, and helps people all over the world with her online classes and individualized services. Contact her for further information: ariele@comcast.net.